Created by <u>BabyDreamers.net</u>

Free Book Offer:

<u>Get How to be a Super Mom For Free</u>

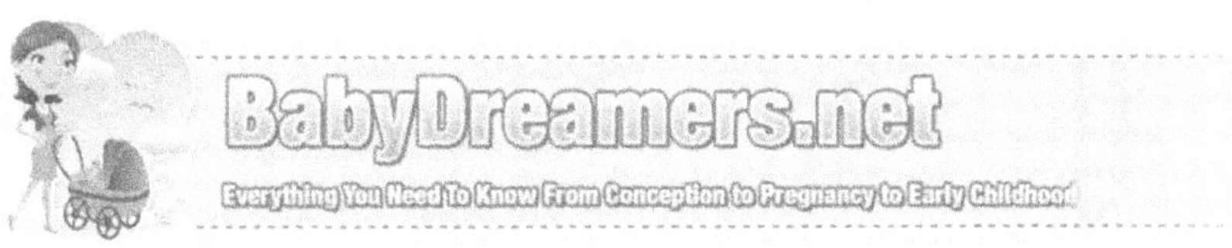

A Short Read is a type of book that is designed to be read in one quick sitting.

These no fluff books are perfect for people who want an overview about a subject in a short period of time.

Table of Contents

The Dos and Don'ts of Trying to Conceive

The journey of trying to conceive a baby can be both exciting and challenging for couples. It is a time filled with hope, anticipation, and sometimes, frustration. To increase your chances of conception, it is important to be aware of the dos and don'ts that can impact fertility. Here are some important tips and advice for couples who are trying to conceive:

- **Do maintain a healthy lifestyle:** Your overall health and well-being play a crucial role in fertility. Make sure to eat a balanced diet, exercise regularly, and avoid harmful substances such as smoking, excessive alcohol consumption, and illicit drugs.
- **Do understand your menstrual cycle:** Knowing your menstrual cycle and when you are most fertile can greatly increase your chances of conceiving. Keep track of your menstrual periods, monitor changes in cervical mucus, and consider using ovulation prediction kits to pinpoint your fertile days.
- **Do have regular and frequent intercourse:** To maximize your chances of getting pregnant, it is recommended to have regular intercourse throughout your menstrual cycle. Aim for at

least two to three times a week to ensure that sperm are present during ovulation.

- **Don't stress too much:** Stress can have a negative impact on fertility. Try to manage stress through relaxation techniques, exercise, and engaging in activities that bring you joy. Consider seeking support from your partner, friends, or joining support groups for individuals struggling with fertility.
- **Don't expose yourself to toxins:** Minimize your exposure to chemicals and environmental toxins that can potentially harm fertility. Be cautious of certain household cleaning products, pesticides, and chemicals found in everyday items.
- **Don't forget about regular check-ups:** It is important to schedule routine medical evaluations for both partners to ensure that any underlying health issues are addressed. Your healthcare provider can offer guidance and support throughout your journey to conceive.

By following these dos and don'ts, you can optimize your chances of conceiving a baby. Remember, every couple's journey is unique, and it may take time and patience. Stay positive, communicate with your partner, and seek professional help if needed. Good luck on your journey to parenthood!

Healthy Lifestyle Choices

When it comes to trying to conceive, making healthy lifestyle choices plays a crucial role in optimizing fertility. A balanced diet, regular exercise, and avoiding harmful substances can all contribute to increasing the chances of conception.

Diet: A nutritious diet rich in fruits, vegetables, whole grains, and lean proteins can provide the essential nutrients needed for reproductive health. Certain foods, such as those high in antioxidants and omega-3 fatty acids, have been linked to improved fertility. It is also important to stay hydrated and limit the consumption of processed foods, sugary drinks, and caffeine.

Exercise: Regular physical activity not only helps maintain a healthy weight but also improves blood circulation and reduces stress levels. Engaging in moderate exercise, such as brisk walking, swimming, or cycling, can have positive effects on reproductive health. However, it is important to avoid excessive exercise, as it may disrupt hormonal balance and affect fertility.

Avoiding Harmful Substances: Smoking, excessive alcohol consumption, and illicit drug use can all have detrimental effects on fertility. These substances can disrupt hormone production, damage reproductive organs, and decrease sperm quality. It is crucial for both partners to refrain from these harmful habits when trying to conceive.

In addition to these lifestyle choices, it is also important to maintain a healthy weight. Obesity and being underweight can both negatively impact fertility. Achieving a healthy weight through a balanced diet and regular exercise can help regulate hormone levels and improve overall reproductive health.

By making these healthy lifestyle choices, couples can create an optimal environment for conception and increase their chances of successfully conceiving a baby.

Timing Intercourse

Timing intercourse is a crucial factor when trying to conceive. Understanding the menstrual cycle and knowing the best time to have sex can greatly increase the chances of conception. The menstrual cycle is divided into different phases, each with its own characteristics and hormonal changes.

One of the key phases to be aware of is ovulation, which is when the egg is released from the ovary and is ready for fertilization. Ovulation typically occurs around the middle of the menstrual cycle, but it can vary from woman to woman. By tracking ovulation, either through methods such as charting basal body temperature or using ovulation predictor kits, couples can identify the most fertile days.

During ovulation, the chances of getting pregnant are highest. Sperm can survive in the female reproductive system for several days, so having sex a few days before ovulation and on the day of ovulation itself can optimize the chances of fertilization. It's important to note that sperm can live inside the female body for up to five days, while the egg is only viable for about 24 hours after ovulation.

For couples trying to conceive, it is recommended to have regular intercourse every two to three days throughout the menstrual cycle. This ensures that sperm are present in the reproductive system during the fertile window, increasing the likelihood of fertilization. However, it's important not to put too much pressure on timing intercourse perfectly, as stress can negatively impact fertility.

In conclusion, understanding the menstrual cycle and timing intercourse accordingly is essential for couples trying to conceive. By tracking ovulation and having regular intercourse, couples can maximize their chances of getting pregnant. Remember to approach the process with patience and a relaxed mindset, as stress can hinder fertility. Good luck on your journey to parenthood!

Tracking Ovulation

Tracking ovulation is an essential step for couples trying to conceive. By understanding when ovulation occurs, couples can time intercourse to increase their chances of getting pregnant. There are several methods and tools available to help determine when ovulation is taking place.

One popular method is tracking changes in cervical mucus. As a woman approaches ovulation, her cervical mucus becomes clear, slippery, and stretchy, resembling the consistency of raw egg whites. By monitoring these changes, couples can identify the most fertile days of the menstrual cycle.

Another method is using ovulation predictor kits (OPKs). These kits detect the surge in luteinizing hormone (LH) that occurs right before ovulation. By testing urine samples, couples can pinpoint the optimal time for intercourse.

Basal body temperature (BBT) tracking is also commonly used. This involves taking the body's temperature every morning before getting out of bed. A slight increase in temperature indicates that ovulation has occurred. By charting these temperatures over time, couples can identify patterns and predict future ovulation.

In addition to these methods, there are also smartphone apps and online tools available that can help track ovulation. These tools often combine multiple methods, such as tracking menstrual cycles, cervical mucus changes, and BBT, to provide a comprehensive overview of fertility.

It's important to note that tracking ovulation is not foolproof and may not work for everyone. Factors such as irregular menstrual cycles or underlying health conditions can affect the accuracy of these methods. If couples are having difficulty determining when ovulation occurs or are experiencing infertility, it is recommended to seek medical advice from a healthcare professional.

Frequency of Intercourse

When it comes to trying to conceive, the frequency of intercourse plays a crucial role in maximizing the chances of getting pregnant. But how often should couples have sex? Is there a magic number that guarantees success?

While there is no one-size-fits-all answer to this question, experts recommend aiming for regular sexual activity throughout the menstrual cycle. This means having sex every 2 to 3 days to ensure that sperm is consistently present in the reproductive system, ready to fertilize the egg when ovulation occurs.

It's important to note that having sex too frequently or too infrequently can both have an impact on fertility. Having sex too often may result in a lower sperm count, as the body needs time to replenish sperm levels. On the other hand, not having sex frequently enough may reduce the chances of sperm meeting the egg during the fertile window.

Understanding the menstrual cycle can also help determine the optimal frequency of intercourse. The fertile window, which is the period when a woman is most likely to conceive, typically occurs around 12 to 16 days before the start of the next menstrual period. Having sex during this time increases the likelihood of pregnancy.

It's worth noting that stress and pressure to conceive can also affect sexual desire and performance. It's important for couples to communicate openly and support each other emotionally throughout the process. Remember, trying to conceive should be an enjoyable and intimate experience for both partners.

In summary, the frequency of intercourse should be regular throughout the menstrual cycle, with a focus on the fertile window. Aim for sex every 2 to 3 days to ensure a consistent supply of sperm. And most importantly, don't forget to relax, enjoy the journey, and prioritize emotional well-being.

Understanding Fertility Issues

Understanding fertility issues is crucial for couples who are trying to conceive. Infertility is defined as the inability to conceive after one year of regular unprotected intercourse. While it can be a challenging and emotionally draining journey, it's important to remember that you are not alone. Many couples face fertility issues, and there are various causes that can contribute to difficulties in conceiving.

Some common causes of infertility include:

- Age-related factors: As a woman ages, her fertility naturally declines. The quality and quantity of eggs decrease, making it more difficult to conceive. It's important to be aware of the impact of age on fertility and seek medical help if you're struggling to conceive.
- Hormonal imbalances: Hormonal imbalances can disrupt the menstrual cycle and interfere with ovulation. Conditions such as polycystic ovary syndrome (PCOS) and thyroid disorders can affect fertility. Seeking medical help and

getting proper diagnosis and treatment is essential in such cases.

- Structural abnormalities: Structural abnormalities in the reproductive organs, such as blocked fallopian tubes or uterine fibroids, can hinder the fertilization process. Medical interventions may be necessary to address these issues.
- Male factor infertility: Infertility is not solely a female issue. Male factors, such as low sperm count or poor sperm motility, can also contribute to difficulties in conceiving. It's important for both partners to undergo fertility evaluations.
- Unhealthy lifestyle choices: Certain lifestyle factors, such as smoking, excessive alcohol consumption, and obesity, can negatively impact fertility. Making healthy choices and adopting a balanced lifestyle can improve your chances of conceiving.

If you and your partner have been actively trying to conceive for a year without success, it may be time to seek medical help. Your healthcare provider can conduct fertility evaluations to identify any underlying issues and recommend appropriate treatments. Remember, early intervention can often lead to successful outcomes.

Age and Fertility

Age plays a crucial role in female fertility. As women age, their fertility naturally decreases. This is because women are born with a finite number of eggs, and as they get older, the quality and quantity of these eggs decline. It is important for women to be aware of how age can impact their ability to conceive and make informed decisions about family planning.

Table: Age and Fertility

Age Range	Fertility Status
20-24	High fertility
25-29	High fertility
30-34	Good fertility
35-39	Decreased fertility
40 and above	Significantly decreased fertility

As shown in the table above, a woman's fertility is generally highest in her early to mid-20s and starts to decline after the age of 30. By the age of 35, fertility significantly decreases, and the chances of conceiving naturally decrease even further as a woman enters her 40s.

It's important to note that while age primarily affects female fertility, it can also impact male fertility to some extent. Advanced paternal age has been associated with a higher risk of certain genetic disorders and a decrease in sperm quality. However, the decline in male fertility with age is generally less pronounced compared to females.

Ultimately, age is a critical factor to consider when trying to conceive. If you are in your late 30s or 40s and struggling to get pregnant, it is advisable to seek medical advice and explore fertility treatments such as in vitro fertilization (IVF) or other assisted reproductive technologies. Understanding the relationship between age and fertility can help individuals make informed decisions and take appropriate steps to maximize their chances of conceiving.

Male Fertility Factors

Male fertility factors play a crucial role in the journey of trying to conceive. While much of the focus is often on female fertility, it is important to recognize that male factors can also significantly impact the chances of conception. Understanding and addressing these factors can greatly improve the chances of successfully achieving pregnancy.

One of the key factors in male fertility is the quality and quantity of sperm. A low sperm count or poor sperm motility can make it more difficult for sperm to reach and fertilize an egg. Lifestyle choices such as smoking, excessive alcohol consumption, and drug use can negatively affect sperm quality. Additionally, certain medical conditions such as varicocele or hormonal imbalances can also contribute to male fertility issues.

To address potential male fertility issues, it is important for men to make healthy lifestyle choices. This includes maintaining a balanced diet rich in nutrients that support reproductive health. Incorporating foods high in antioxidants, such as fruits and vegetables, can help protect sperm from oxidative damage. Regular exercise and maintaining a healthy weight are also beneficial for overall reproductive health.

In addition to lifestyle changes, there are other steps that can be taken to address male fertility issues. If a man suspects he may have a medical condition impacting fertility, it is important to seek medical advice and undergo necessary tests. Treatment options may include medication, surgery, or assisted reproductive techniques such as intrauterine insemination (IUI) or in vitro fertilization (IVF).

Furthermore, it can be helpful for couples to track the woman's menstrual cycle and time intercourse accordingly. Having sex during the woman's fertile window, which typically occurs around ovulation, can increase the chances of conception. There are various methods and tools available to help determine when ovulation is likely to occur, such as ovulation predictor kits or tracking basal body temperature.

In conclusion, male fertility factors play a significant role in the journey of trying to conceive. By addressing potential issues and making healthy lifestyle choices, couples can increase their chances of successfully achieving pregnancy. Seeking medical advice when necessary and understanding the woman's menstrual cycle can also help optimize the timing of intercourse. Remember, both partners' reproductive health is essential in the quest to start a family.

Creating a Healthy Environment

Creating a healthy environment is crucial for optimizing the reproductive environment and increasing the chances of conception. Here are some tips to help couples create the ideal conditions for fertility:

- **Maintain a balanced diet:** A nutritious diet plays a vital role in reproductive health. Include a variety of fruits, vegetables, whole grains, lean proteins, and healthy fats in your diet. Avoid processed foods, excessive caffeine, and alcohol, as they can negatively impact fertility.
- **Stay hydrated:** Drinking an adequate amount of water is essential for overall health, including reproductive health. Aim to drink at least 8 glasses of water per day.
- **Manage weight:** Maintaining a healthy weight is important for both men and women when trying to conceive. Being overweight or underweight can affect hormone levels and disrupt the menstrual cycle.
- **Exercise regularly:** Engaging in moderate exercise can improve blood circulation, reduce stress, and promote hormonal balance. However, avoid excessive exercise, as it may have a negative impact on fertility.
- **Avoid exposure to toxins:** Minimize exposure to harmful chemicals, such as pesticides,

household cleaning products, and certain beauty products. Opt for natural and organic alternatives whenever possible.
- **Get enough sleep:** A good night's sleep is essential for overall well-being and reproductive health. Aim for 7-8 hours of quality sleep each night.
- **Reduce stress:** High levels of stress can interfere with fertility. Find healthy ways to manage stress, such as practicing relaxation techniques, engaging in hobbies, or seeking support from loved ones.
- **Consider environmental factors:** Create a conducive environment for conception by ensuring the bedroom is cool, well-ventilated, and free from distractions. Avoid excessive exposure to electromagnetic radiation from electronic devices.

By implementing these tips, couples can optimize their reproductive environment and increase their chances of conceiving a baby. It's important to remember that creating a healthy environment is a joint effort that requires both partners to make lifestyle changes and support each other throughout the journey.

Managing Stress

Managing stress is crucial for couples who are trying to conceive, as stress can have a significant impact on fertility. When the body is under stress, it releases cortisol, a hormone that can interfere with the reproductive system. High levels of cortisol can disrupt the delicate hormonal balance necessary for ovulation and implantation.

Fortunately, there are several coping strategies that couples can employ to reduce stress and increase their chances of conceiving. One effective method is to practice relaxation techniques such as deep breathing, meditation, or yoga. These activities can help calm the mind and body, reducing stress levels and promoting overall well-being.

Another way to manage stress is to engage in regular exercise. Physical activity releases endorphins, also known as "feel-good" hormones, which can help alleviate stress and improve mood. Whether it's going for a walk, participating in a fitness class, or engaging in a favorite sport, finding an exercise routine that suits both partners can be beneficial for reducing stress and enhancing fertility.

In addition to relaxation techniques and exercise, it's important for couples to communicate openly and support each other during the trying-to-conceive journey. Sharing feelings, concerns, and frustrations can help alleviate stress and strengthen the bond between partners. It may also be helpful to seek support from friends, family, or a professional counselor who specializes in fertility issues.

Creating a peaceful and nurturing environment at home can also contribute to stress reduction. Couples can consider setting aside time for activities they enjoy together, such as taking walks in nature, cooking healthy meals, or practicing hobbies. Creating a positive and harmonious atmosphere can help alleviate stress and promote a sense of well-being.

Lastly, it's important for couples to remember that trying to conceive is a journey that requires patience and resilience. It's normal to feel stressed or anxious at times, but it's essential to focus on self-care and maintaining a positive mindset. Taking breaks, engaging in activities that bring joy, and practicing self-compassion can all contribute to managing stress and increasing fertility.

Avoiding Toxins

Avoiding toxins is an important aspect of optimizing fertility and increasing the chances of conception. Chemicals and environmental toxins can have a negative impact on reproductive health, affecting both male and female fertility. It is crucial to identify these toxins and take steps to minimize exposure to them.

One of the first steps in avoiding toxins is to be aware of the potential sources of chemicals and environmental toxins. These can include household cleaning products, pesticides, certain cosmetics and personal care products, and even certain types of food. By reading labels and being mindful of the ingredients in these products, you can make informed choices and opt for safer alternatives.

In addition to being cautious about the products you use, it is important to minimize exposure to environmental toxins. This can include avoiding smoking and secondhand smoke, as well as limiting exposure to air pollution and certain chemicals found in workplaces or industrial areas. Taking steps to improve indoor air quality, such as using air purifiers and ensuring proper ventilation, can also help reduce exposure to toxins.

Creating a healthy environment for conception also involves making lifestyle changes. Eating a nutritious diet rich in fruits, vegetables, whole grains, and lean proteins can support overall health and fertility. Choosing organic produce and opting for hormone-free meat and dairy products can also reduce exposure to pesticides and hormones that may affect reproductive health.

It is also important to stay hydrated by drinking plenty of water and to engage in regular exercise. Exercise helps maintain a healthy weight, improves circulation, and reduces stress, all of which can positively impact fertility. However, it is important to avoid excessive exercise, as this can also have a negative effect on reproductive health.

In conclusion, avoiding toxins is a crucial step in optimizing fertility. By identifying and minimizing exposure to chemicals and environmental toxins, couples can create a healthier environment for conception. Being mindful of the products used, making lifestyle changes, and taking steps to reduce exposure to toxins can all contribute to improving reproductive health and increasing the chances of successfully conceiving a baby.

Optimizing Reproductive Health

Optimizing reproductive health is crucial for couples who are trying to conceive. By taking proactive steps to improve overall reproductive health, both partners can increase their chances of achieving a successful pregnancy. Here are some important steps to consider:

- **Healthy Diet:** Eating a balanced diet rich in fruits, vegetables, whole grains, and lean proteins can provide essential nutrients that support reproductive health. It's also important to stay hydrated and limit the consumption of processed foods and sugary beverages.
- **Regular Exercise:** Engaging in regular physical activity can help maintain a healthy weight and improve blood circulation, which is beneficial for reproductive health. Aim for at least 30 minutes of moderate exercise most days of the week.
- **Avoiding Harmful Substances:** Smoking, excessive alcohol consumption, and illicit drug use can all negatively impact fertility. It's important for both partners to avoid these substances to optimize reproductive health.
- **Manage Stress:** High levels of stress can interfere with hormone production and disrupt the menstrual cycle. Finding healthy ways to manage stress, such as through exercise, meditation, or engaging in hobbies, can help support reproductive health.

- **Get Enough Sleep:** A good night's sleep is essential for overall health, including reproductive health. Aim for 7-9 hours of quality sleep each night to support hormonal balance and overall well-being.
- **Limit Exposure to Environmental Toxins:** Certain chemicals and toxins found in everyday products can have a negative impact on reproductive health. Minimize exposure to pesticides, household cleaning products, and plastics that contain harmful chemicals.
- **Manage Chronic Conditions:** If you or your partner have any chronic health conditions, it's important to work with your healthcare provider to manage them effectively. Conditions such as diabetes, thyroid disorders, and autoimmune diseases can affect fertility.

By incorporating these steps into your lifestyle, you can optimize your reproductive health and increase your chances of conceiving a baby. Remember, it's important to consult with a healthcare professional for personalized advice and guidance based on your specific needs and circumstances.

Importance of Regular Check-ups

Regular check-ups are an essential aspect of maintaining reproductive health and increasing the chances of conceiving. These routine medical evaluations provide numerous benefits for couples who are trying to conceive. By scheduling regular check-ups, individuals can proactively address any potential fertility issues and take necessary steps to optimize their reproductive health.

One of the primary benefits of regular check-ups is the opportunity to identify and address any underlying medical conditions that may be affecting fertility. During these evaluations, healthcare professionals can perform comprehensive examinations and tests to assess the overall reproductive health of both partners. They can identify any potential obstacles to conception, such as hormonal imbalances or structural abnormalities, and recommend appropriate treatments or interventions.

In addition to diagnosing and treating fertility-related conditions, regular check-ups also offer a chance to monitor the progress of any ongoing treatments or interventions. Healthcare professionals can track the effectiveness of medications or procedures and make adjustments as necessary. This ongoing monitoring ensures that couples are on the right path towards achieving their goal of conceiving a baby.

Furthermore, regular check-ups provide an opportunity for couples to receive guidance and support from knowledgeable healthcare professionals. These professionals can offer advice on lifestyle modifications, such as diet and exercise, that can enhance fertility. They can also provide information on the latest advancements in reproductive medicine and assist couples in making informed decisions about their fertility journey.

Ultimately, regular check-ups play a crucial role in maintaining and improving fertility. By prioritizing these routine medical evaluations, couples can take proactive steps towards optimizing their reproductive health and increasing their chances of conceiving a baby.

Supplements and Vitamins

Supplements and vitamins play a crucial role in supporting fertility for both men and women. They can help optimize reproductive health, address any nutrient deficiencies, and enhance the chances of conceiving a baby. It is important to note that while supplements and vitamins can be beneficial, they should never replace a healthy diet and lifestyle.

For women, certain vitamins and minerals are particularly important for fertility. These include folic acid, which helps prevent neural tube defects in the developing baby, and iron, which supports healthy blood production. Omega-3 fatty acids, found in fish oil supplements, have also been shown to improve fertility by promoting hormonal balance and reducing inflammation.

For men, supplements can also play a role in improving fertility. Zinc is a key mineral that supports sperm production and motility. Coenzyme Q10 (CoQ10) is an antioxidant that helps protect sperm from oxidative damage. Additionally, vitamin C and vitamin E have been shown to improve sperm quality and function.

It is important to consult with a healthcare professional before starting any supplements or vitamins, as they can interact with medications or have potential side effects. They can also help determine the appropriate dosage and duration of supplementation.

Remember, supplements and vitamins should always be used as a complement to a healthy diet and lifestyle. Eating a balanced diet rich in fruits, vegetables, whole grains, lean proteins, and healthy fats is essential for overall reproductive health. Regular exercise, maintaining a healthy weight, and managing stress are also important factors to consider when trying to conceive.

In summary, supplements and vitamins can play a supportive role in fertility by addressing nutrient deficiencies and optimizing reproductive health. However, it is important to consult with a healthcare professional and prioritize a healthy lifestyle for the best chances of conceiving a baby.

Understanding the Menstrual Cycle

The menstrual cycle is a natural process that occurs in the female reproductive system. It involves a series of hormonal changes and physical events that prepare the body for pregnancy. Understanding the different phases of the menstrual cycle is essential for couples who are trying to conceive.

The menstrual cycle is typically divided into four phases: the menstrual phase, the follicular phase, the ovulatory phase, and the luteal phase. Let's take a closer look at each phase:

- **Menstrual Phase:** This is the first phase of the menstrual cycle and is characterized by the shedding of the uterine lining. It usually lasts for about 3 to 7 days and is accompanied by menstrual bleeding. During this phase, hormone levels are low, and the body prepares for the next phase.
- **Follicular Phase:** The follicular phase begins immediately after the menstrual phase and lasts for about 7 to 10 days. During this phase, the pituitary gland releases follicle-stimulating hormone (FSH), which stimulates the development of follicles in the ovaries. These follicles contain eggs, and as they grow, they release estrogen, which thickens the uterine lining.
- **Ovulatory Phase:** The ovulatory phase is the shortest phase of the menstrual cycle, lasting only about 24 to 48 hours. It occurs when a mature egg is released from one of the follicles in the ovaries. This process is triggered by a surge in luteinizing hormone (LH) and is essential for conception. The egg travels through the fallopian tubes, where it can be fertilized by sperm.

- **Luteal Phase:** The luteal phase begins after ovulation and lasts for about 10 to 14 days. During this phase, the ruptured follicle in the ovary transforms into a structure called the corpus luteum, which produces progesterone. Progesterone helps thicken the uterine lining and prepare it for implantation. If fertilization does not occur, hormone levels drop, and the uterine lining is shed, marking the start of a new menstrual cycle.

Tracking the menstrual cycle and understanding its phases can help couples identify the most fertile days for conception. Ovulation typically occurs around the middle of the menstrual cycle, so timing intercourse during this period can increase the chances of pregnancy. There are various methods and tools available to track ovulation, such as ovulation predictor kits and tracking basal body temperature.

It's important to note that every woman's menstrual cycle may vary in length and regularity. Factors such as stress, illness, and hormonal imbalances can affect the timing and duration of each phase. If you have concerns about your menstrual cycle or are experiencing difficulties conceiving, it is recommended to consult with a healthcare professional.

Menstrual Cycle Disorders

Menstrual cycle disorders are common conditions that can significantly impact fertility. These disorders refer to any abnormalities or irregularities in the menstrual cycle, including changes in the frequency, duration, or intensity of periods. Understanding these disorders and their treatment options is crucial for couples trying to conceive.

One common menstrual cycle disorder is Polycystic Ovary Syndrome (PCOS). PCOS is characterized by hormonal imbalances that can disrupt ovulation and lead to irregular or absent periods. This condition affects approximately 1 in 10 women of reproductive age and can make it more challenging to conceive. Treatment options for PCOS may include lifestyle changes, such as weight loss and exercise, as well as medications to regulate hormone levels and induce ovulation.

Another disorder that can affect fertility is endometriosis. Endometriosis occurs when the tissue that lines the uterus grows outside of the uterus, often causing pain and inflammation. This condition can interfere with the release of eggs and the implantation of a fertilized egg. Treatment options for endometriosis may include pain management medications, hormone therapy, or surgery to remove the abnormal tissue.

Other menstrual cycle disorders that can impact fertility include irregular periods, amenorrhea (absence of periods), and dysmenorrhea (painful periods). These disorders can be caused by various factors, such as hormonal imbalances, thyroid disorders, or structural abnormalities in the reproductive organs. Treatment options for these disorders depend on the underlying cause and may involve hormonal medications, lifestyle changes, or surgical interventions.

It is essential for individuals experiencing menstrual cycle disorders to consult with a healthcare professional specializing in reproductive health. They can provide a proper diagnosis, discuss treatment options, and offer guidance on optimizing fertility. By addressing these disorders, couples can increase their chances of conceiving and starting a family.

Basal Body Temperature Tracking

Basal Body Temperature (BBT) tracking is a method used by many couples to monitor the menstrual cycle and predict ovulation. This technique involves measuring the body's lowest resting temperature, which is known as the basal body temperature. By tracking these temperature changes over time, couples can gain valuable insights into their fertility and increase their chances of conception.

To start tracking your basal body temperature, you will need a special thermometer designed for this purpose. It is important to measure your temperature at the same time every morning, before engaging in any physical activity or even getting out of bed. This consistency ensures accurate and reliable results.

Once you have recorded your temperature for several cycles, you can start to observe patterns and identify the rise in temperature that indicates ovulation. Typically, a woman's basal body temperature will be lower in the first half of her menstrual cycle and then rise by about 0.5 to 1 degree Fahrenheit after ovulation.

It is important to note that basal body temperature tracking alone is not foolproof in predicting ovulation. Other signs and symptoms, such as changes in cervical mucus and the position of the cervix, should also be considered. Additionally, factors such as illness, lack of sleep, and alcohol consumption can affect basal body temperature readings.

By combining basal body temperature tracking with other methods, such as monitoring cervical mucus and using ovulation predictor kits, couples can gain a more comprehensive understanding of their fertility and increase their chances of conceiving.

Healthy Habits for Men

When it comes to trying to conceive, it's not just the women who need to make healthy lifestyle choices. Men play an equally important role in fertility, and there are specific habits they can adopt to improve their chances of conception. Here are some healthy habits for men that can enhance male fertility:

- **Diet and Nutrition:** A balanced diet rich in fruits, vegetables, whole grains, lean proteins, and healthy fats can positively impact sperm quality. Certain nutrients like zinc, selenium, vitamin C, and antioxidants are particularly beneficial for fertility. It's also important to stay hydrated and limit the consumption of processed foods, sugary drinks, and excessive alcohol.

- **Exercise and Physical Activity:** Regular exercise not only helps maintain a healthy weight but also improves blood circulation, which is crucial for reproductive health. Engaging in moderate-intensity exercises like jogging, swimming, or cycling can boost sperm production and motility. However, it's important to avoid excessive physical activity, as it may have a negative impact on fertility.
- **Avoiding Environmental Toxins:** Exposure to certain chemicals and toxins can harm sperm quality and fertility. Men should minimize their exposure to pesticides, heavy metals, and harmful substances like tobacco, drugs, and excessive heat. It's advisable to wear protective clothing and follow safety guidelines when working with chemicals or in high-temperature environments.
- **Stress Management:** Chronic stress can affect hormone levels and sperm production. Finding healthy ways to manage stress, such as practicing relaxation techniques, engaging in hobbies, or seeking support from loved ones, can have a positive impact on male fertility.

- **Adequate Sleep:** Getting enough sleep is essential for overall health, including reproductive health. Lack of sleep can disrupt hormone production and affect sperm quality. Aim for 7-8 hours of quality sleep each night to support optimal fertility.
- **Maintaining a Healthy Weight:** Obesity and being underweight can both negatively impact male fertility. It's important to maintain a healthy weight through a balanced diet and regular exercise. Consulting with a healthcare professional or a registered dietitian can help develop a personalized plan.
- **Avoiding Excessive Heat:** High temperatures can hinder sperm production. Men should avoid hot tubs, saunas, and tight-fitting underwear to keep the testicles cool and promote healthy sperm production.

By adopting these healthy habits, men can take an active role in optimizing their fertility and increasing the chances of successfully conceiving a baby. It's important for couples to work together as a team and support each other throughout the journey of trying to conceive.

Diet and Nutrition for Men

Diet plays a crucial role in maintaining overall health and well-being, and it also has a significant impact on sperm quality and fertility in men. Consuming a balanced and nutritious diet can help optimize reproductive health and increase the chances of conception. Here are some key dietary recommendations for men who are trying to conceive:

- **Increase intake of fruits and vegetables:** Fresh fruits and vegetables are rich in antioxidants and essential nutrients that can improve sperm health. Aim for a variety of colorful fruits and vegetables to ensure a wide range of nutrients.
- **Choose lean protein sources:** Opt for lean meats, poultry, fish, and plant-based protein sources such as beans and lentils. These protein-rich foods provide essential amino acids that are important for sperm production.
- **Include healthy fats:** Incorporate sources of healthy fats into your diet, such as avocados, nuts, seeds, and olive oil. These fats contain omega-3 fatty acids, which are beneficial for sperm quality.
- **Avoid excessive alcohol consumption:** Excessive alcohol intake can negatively affect sperm production and quality. It's best to limit alcohol consumption or avoid it altogether when trying to conceive.
- **Reduce caffeine intake:** High caffeine intake has been associated with reduced fertility in

men. Limit your consumption of coffee, tea, energy drinks, and other caffeinated beverages.

- **Stay hydrated:** Drinking an adequate amount of water is essential for overall health, including reproductive health. Aim to drink at least 8 glasses of water per day.
- **Limit processed and sugary foods:** Processed foods and foods high in added sugars can contribute to inflammation and negatively impact sperm quality. Opt for whole, unprocessed foods whenever possible.
- **Consider supplementation:** In addition to a healthy diet, certain supplements may be beneficial for male fertility. Talk to your healthcare provider about potential supplements such as zinc, selenium, and coenzyme Q10.

Remember, maintaining a healthy diet is just one aspect of optimizing fertility in men. It's also important to lead a healthy lifestyle overall, which includes regular exercise, managing stress levels, and avoiding harmful substances. By making positive lifestyle choices and paying attention to nutrition, men can enhance their reproductive health and increase their chances of successfully conceiving with their partner.

Exercise and Male Fertility

Exercise plays a crucial role in maintaining overall health and well-being, and it also has a significant impact on male fertility. Regular physical activity can improve sperm quality, increase sperm count, and enhance reproductive function in men.

Engaging in moderate-intensity exercise, such as brisk walking, jogging, or cycling, can boost blood flow to the reproductive organs and promote the production of healthy sperm. It helps to improve hormonal balance, reduce oxidative stress, and enhance the body's ability to eliminate toxins, all of which contribute to better reproductive health.

However, it is important to note that excessive exercise or intense physical training can have a negative impact on male fertility. Overtraining and excessive physical exertion can lead to hormonal imbalances, decreased sperm production, and even erectile dysfunction. Therefore, finding a balance and avoiding extreme exercise routines is essential.

In addition to cardiovascular exercises, incorporating strength training into your fitness routine can also benefit male fertility. Resistance training helps to increase testosterone levels, which is crucial for sperm production. It can also improve muscle mass and overall body composition, leading to better reproductive health.

It is important to consult with a healthcare professional or a fertility specialist to determine the appropriate level of exercise for your individual needs. They can provide guidance on the duration, intensity, and type of exercises that are most beneficial for male fertility.

In summary, regular exercise is beneficial for male fertility, but moderation is key. Engaging in moderate-intensity exercises, such as cardio and strength training, can improve sperm quality and reproductive function. However, excessive exercise or intense physical training can have a negative impact on fertility. Finding a balance and consulting with a healthcare professional is crucial to optimize male reproductive health.

Addressing Medical Conditions

Addressing Medical Conditions

When it comes to trying to conceive, certain medical conditions can have a significant impact on fertility. Understanding these conditions and exploring potential treatment options is crucial for couples who are struggling to get pregnant. Here, we will discuss some common medical conditions that can affect fertility and the steps that can be taken to address them.

Polycystic Ovary Syndrome (PCOS):

PCOS is a hormonal disorder that affects women of reproductive age. It can disrupt the normal ovulation process, making it difficult to conceive. Women with PCOS may experience irregular periods, excess hair growth, and cysts on their ovaries. Treatment options for PCOS may include lifestyle changes, such as maintaining a healthy weight and managing insulin levels, as well as medications to regulate ovulation.

Endometriosis:

Endometriosis is a condition in which the tissue that normally lines the uterus grows outside of it. This can cause inflammation, scarring, and the formation of adhesions, which can interfere with fertility. Women with endometriosis may experience pelvic pain, heavy periods, and difficulty getting pregnant. Treatment options for endometriosis may include medication to manage symptoms, surgery to remove abnormal tissue, or assisted reproductive technologies (ART) like in vitro fertilization (IVF).

By addressing these medical conditions and seeking appropriate treatment, couples can increase their chances of conceiving and starting a family. It is important to consult with a healthcare professional who specializes in fertility to determine the best course of action based on individual circumstances.

Polycystic Ovary Syndrome (PCOS)

Polycystic Ovary Syndrome (PCOS) is a hormonal disorder that affects women of reproductive age. It is characterized by the presence of multiple cysts on the ovaries, irregular menstrual cycles, and high levels of androgens (male hormones) in the body. PCOS can have a significant impact on fertility and make it more challenging for women to conceive.

One of the main effects of PCOS on fertility is the disruption of ovulation. Women with PCOS often experience irregular or absent menstrual periods, which means that they may not release an egg every month. Without regular ovulation, the chances of getting pregnant naturally are reduced.

Managing PCOS and improving fertility often involves a combination of lifestyle changes, medication, and fertility treatments. Women with PCOS are often advised to maintain a healthy weight through diet and exercise, as excess weight can exacerbate hormonal imbalances and make it more difficult to conceive. It is also important to avoid smoking and limit alcohol consumption, as these can further disrupt hormone levels.

In some cases, medication may be prescribed to regulate the menstrual cycle and induce ovulation. Commonly used medications include clomiphene citrate and letrozole, which help stimulate the ovaries to release eggs. In more severe cases, assisted reproductive technologies such as in vitro fertilization (IVF) may be recommended.

It is important for women with PCOS to work closely with their healthcare provider to develop a personalized treatment plan that addresses their specific needs and goals. Regular monitoring of hormone levels and ultrasound examinations may be necessary to track progress and adjust treatment as needed.

Overall, while PCOS can present challenges when it comes to fertility, there are various strategies and treatments available to help manage the condition and increase the chances of conceiving. With the right support and guidance, women with PCOS can navigate the journey of trying to conceive and fulfill their dreams of starting a family.

Endometriosis

Endometriosis is a condition that can have a significant impact on fertility. It occurs when the tissue that normally lines the uterus, called the endometrium, starts growing outside of the uterus. This abnormal growth can affect the function of the reproductive organs and make it more difficult for a woman to conceive.

One of the main ways endometriosis can affect fertility is by causing the formation of scar tissue. As the endometrial tissue grows in places it shouldn't, it can create adhesions and scar tissue that can distort the reproductive organs. This can lead to blockages in the fallopian tubes or the ovaries, making it difficult for the egg to travel to the uterus or for the sperm to reach the egg.

Another way endometriosis can impact fertility is by causing inflammation. The presence of endometrial tissue outside of the uterus can trigger an immune response, leading to inflammation in the pelvic region. This inflammation can affect the quality of the eggs and sperm, making fertilization less likely to occur.

Fortunately, there are treatment options available for women with endometriosis who are trying to conceive. One common approach is laparoscopic surgery, which aims to remove the endometrial tissue and any scar tissue or adhesions that may be present. This can help improve fertility by restoring the normal function of the reproductive organs.

In addition to surgery, other treatment options for endometriosis-related infertility include hormonal therapies and assisted reproductive technologies. Hormonal therapies, such as birth control pills or gonadotropin-releasing hormone (GnRH) agonists, can help regulate the menstrual cycle and reduce the growth of endometrial tissue. Assisted reproductive technologies, such as in vitro fertilization (IVF), can bypass any blockages or other issues caused by endometriosis and increase the chances of pregnancy.

It's important for women with endometriosis who are trying to conceive to work closely with their healthcare provider to develop a personalized treatment plan. Each case of endometriosis is unique, and the appropriate treatment approach will depend on factors such as the severity of the condition and the woman's age.

In conclusion, endometriosis can have a significant impact on fertility, but there are treatment options available to help women with this condition conceive. By addressing the underlying causes of infertility and working with a healthcare provider, women with endometriosis can increase their chances of achieving a successful pregnancy.

Alternative Approaches

Alternative Approaches

When it comes to trying to conceive, couples often explore alternative methods and practices that may enhance fertility. While these approaches may not have scientific evidence to support their effectiveness, many individuals have found them to be helpful in their journey towards parenthood. Here are a few alternative approaches that you may consider:

- **Acupuncture and Fertility:** Acupuncture is an ancient Chinese practice that involves inserting thin needles into specific points on the body. Some studies suggest that acupuncture may help improve fertility outcomes by promoting blood flow to the reproductive organs and reducing stress. If you're considering acupuncture, it's important to find a licensed and experienced practitioner.
- **Herbal Remedies:** Certain herbs and natural remedies are believed to support fertility. For example, chasteberry is often used to regulate the menstrual cycle, while maca root is thought to enhance overall reproductive health. However, it's crucial to consult with a healthcare professional before incorporating any herbal remedies into your fertility journey.

It's important to note that alternative approaches should be used in conjunction with evidence-based medical treatments and under the guidance of healthcare professionals. While they may offer additional support, they should not replace conventional medical advice and interventions. Ultimately, the decision to explore alternative approaches is a personal one, and it's essential to prioritize your physical and emotional well-being throughout the process.

Acupuncture and Fertility

Acupuncture has gained popularity as an alternative approach to improving fertility outcomes. This ancient Chinese practice involves the insertion of thin needles into specific points on the body to stimulate energy flow and promote overall well-being. While the exact mechanisms are not fully understood, acupuncture is believed to have several potential benefits for couples trying to conceive.

One of the main ways acupuncture may support fertility is by reducing stress levels. Trying to conceive can be a stressful journey, and stress has been shown to negatively impact fertility. Acupuncture sessions can provide a calming and relaxing experience, helping to alleviate stress and promote emotional well-being. By reducing stress, acupuncture may help regulate hormonal imbalances and improve reproductive function.

In addition to stress reduction, acupuncture may also improve blood flow to the reproductive organs. Proper blood circulation is essential for optimal reproductive health, as it ensures that the ovaries and uterus receive an adequate supply of oxygen and nutrients. By enhancing blood flow, acupuncture may help create a more favorable environment for conception to occur.

Furthermore, acupuncture may have a positive impact on the hormonal balance within the body. Hormonal imbalances can disrupt the menstrual cycle and interfere with ovulation. Acupuncture is believed to regulate hormone levels, promoting regular menstrual cycles and increasing the chances of successful ovulation.

It is important to note that while acupuncture may offer potential benefits for fertility, it is not a standalone solution. It is best used in conjunction with other healthy lifestyle choices and medical interventions, if necessary. Consulting with a qualified acupuncturist who specializes in fertility can provide personalized guidance and treatment plans tailored to individual needs.

In summary, acupuncture has the potential to improve fertility outcomes by reducing stress, enhancing blood flow, and regulating hormonal balance. While further research is needed to fully understand its mechanisms of action, many couples have reported positive experiences with acupuncture as part of their fertility journey. If considering acupuncture as a complementary approach to fertility, it is important to consult with a qualified practitioner and discuss any concerns or questions.

Herbal Remedies

Herbal remedies have been used for centuries to support fertility and enhance reproductive health. While their effectiveness may vary from person to person, many couples turn to these natural remedies as a complementary approach to their journey of trying to conceive.

Here is an overview of some popular herbal remedies that are believed to support fertility:

- **Vitex:** Also known as chasteberry, Vitex is a popular herb that is often used to regulate hormone levels and promote regular menstrual cycles. It is believed to help balance estrogen and progesterone levels, which can be beneficial for women with irregular periods or hormonal imbalances.
- **Maca:** Maca root is a Peruvian herb that is known for its adaptogenic properties. It is believed to help balance hormones, increase libido, and improve overall reproductive health. Maca is often used by both men and women to support fertility.
- **Raspberry Leaf:** Raspberry leaf is commonly used as a uterine tonic and is believed to strengthen the uterus and improve the chances of implantation. It is often consumed as a tea or taken in capsule form.
- **Red Clover:** Red clover is rich in phytoestrogens, which are plant compounds that mimic the effects of estrogen in the body. It is believed to support hormonal balance and improve the quality of cervical mucus, making it easier for sperm to reach the egg.
- **Nettle Leaf:** Nettle leaf is a nutrient-rich herb that is believed to support overall reproductive

health. It is high in vitamins and minerals, including iron, which is important for healthy blood flow and fertility.

It is important to note that while herbal remedies are generally considered safe, it is always recommended to consult with a healthcare professional before incorporating them into your fertility journey. They can provide personalized guidance and ensure that the chosen herbs are suitable for your specific needs and health conditions.

Emotional Support

Emotional support plays a crucial role in the journey of trying to conceive. The process of trying to get pregnant can be emotionally challenging and can take a toll on both individuals in a relationship. It is important to prioritize emotional well-being and establish a support system to navigate the ups and downs of this journey.

One way to find emotional support is by joining support groups specifically designed for individuals struggling with fertility. These groups provide a safe space where individuals can share their experiences, fears, and frustrations with others who are going through similar challenges. Being a part of a support group can offer a sense of belonging and understanding, and it can be comforting to know that you are not alone in this journey.

In addition to support groups, counseling and therapy can also be beneficial for couples trying to conceive. Infertility can cause significant stress, anxiety, and even depression. Seeking professional help can provide couples with the tools and coping strategies to manage these emotions effectively. A therapist can help individuals navigate the complex emotions associated with infertility and provide guidance on how to communicate and support each other throughout the process.

It is important to remember that emotional well-being is just as important as physical health when trying to conceive. Taking care of your emotional needs can contribute to a healthier mindset and overall well-being, which can positively impact your fertility journey. So, don't hesitate to reach out for emotional support and prioritize self-care along the way.

Support Groups

Support groups can be a valuable resource for individuals struggling with fertility issues. These groups provide a safe and supportive environment where individuals can connect with others who are going through similar experiences. By joining a support group, individuals struggling with fertility can find comfort, understanding, and a sense of community.

One of the key benefits of support groups is the opportunity to share experiences and emotions with others who truly understand. Infertility can be a challenging and isolating journey, and it can be difficult for friends and family members to fully comprehend the emotional toll it takes. Support groups offer a space where individuals can openly discuss their feelings, fears, and frustrations without judgment.

Support groups also provide a wealth of information and resources. Members can share their knowledge about various fertility treatments, doctors, and clinics, which can be incredibly helpful for individuals who are just beginning their fertility journey. Additionally, support group facilitators often invite guest speakers, such as fertility specialists or psychologists, to provide expert advice and guidance.

Another benefit of joining a support group is the opportunity to form friendships and build a support network. The connections made in these groups can be long-lasting and provide ongoing support even after individuals achieve their desired outcome. Members often develop close bonds and become a source of strength and encouragement for one another.

In addition to emotional support, support groups can also offer practical advice and coping strategies. Members can share tips for managing stress, navigating the healthcare system, and dealing with the ups and downs of fertility treatments. This exchange of knowledge and experiences can empower individuals and help them feel more in control of their fertility journey.

Overall, support groups play a crucial role in providing emotional support, information, and a sense of community for individuals struggling with fertility. By joining a support group, individuals can find solace in knowing that they are not alone in their journey and gain valuable insights and resources to navigate the challenges of infertility.

Counseling and Therapy

Counseling and therapy play a crucial role in helping couples navigate the emotional challenges that come with infertility. Dealing with the inability to conceive can be an incredibly stressful and disheartening experience, and it is important for couples to have a safe space where they can express their emotions, fears, and frustrations.

Therapy provides couples with the opportunity to explore their feelings and thoughts surrounding infertility in a supportive and non-judgmental environment. A trained therapist can help couples develop coping strategies and provide guidance on how to manage the emotional rollercoaster that often accompanies the journey of trying to conceive.

During counseling sessions, couples can learn effective communication techniques, which can strengthen their relationship and help them navigate the challenges of infertility as a team. The therapist can also provide education and resources about the various treatment options available, helping couples make informed decisions about their reproductive health.

Additionally, therapy can address any underlying issues that may be contributing to the emotional distress experienced by couples. It is not uncommon for infertility to trigger feelings of guilt, shame, or inadequacy. Through therapy, couples can work through these complex emotions and develop a healthier mindset.

Support groups can also be a valuable resource for couples going through infertility. These groups provide a sense of community and understanding, as individuals share their experiences and offer support to one another. Being surrounded by others who are going through similar challenges can provide a sense of validation and reduce feelings of isolation.

In summary, counseling and therapy offer couples a supportive space to process their emotions, develop coping strategies, and strengthen their relationship. By seeking professional help, couples can navigate the emotional challenges of infertility with greater resilience and find the support they need to cope with this difficult journey.

Frequently Asked Questions

- **What lifestyle choices can impact fertility?**

  Maintaining a healthy diet, engaging in regular exercise, and avoiding harmful substances such as smoking and excessive alcohol consumption can all have a positive impact on fertility.

- **How can I track ovulation?**

  There are several methods to track ovulation, including monitoring changes in cervical mucus, using ovulation predictor kits, and tracking basal body temperature. These methods can help you identify your most fertile days.

- **How often should we have intercourse to maximize our chances of getting pregnant?**

It is generally recommended to have intercourse every 2-3 days throughout the menstrual cycle to ensure sperm is present during ovulation. However, it's important to remember that quality is more important than quantity when it comes to sperm.

- **When should we seek medical help for infertility?**

If you have been actively trying to conceive for a year without success (or six months if you're over 35), it may be time to consult with a fertility specialist. They can help identify any underlying issues and recommend appropriate treatments.

- **Does age affect fertility?**

Yes, age can significantly impact female fertility. As women get older, the quality and quantity of their eggs decrease, making it more difficult to conceive. It's important to be aware of the potential challenges and consider seeking help earlier if you're older.

- **What role do male factors play in fertility?**

Male factors, such as sperm count, motility, and morphology, can also affect fertility. It's important for men to maintain a healthy lifestyle, avoid excessive heat exposure, and address any potential issues with a healthcare professional.

- **How can we optimize the reproductive environment for conception?**

Managing stress, avoiding exposure to toxins and chemicals, maintaining a healthy weight, and ensuring both partners are in good overall health can all contribute to creating a favorable reproductive environment.

- **Are there any supplements or vitamins that can support fertility?**

Certain supplements, such as folic acid, vitamin D, and omega-3 fatty acids, have been associated with improved fertility outcomes. However, it's important to consult with a healthcare professional before starting any new supplements.

- **How does stress impact fertility?**

High levels of stress can disrupt hormone balance and interfere with ovulation. Finding healthy ways to manage stress, such as through exercise, relaxation techniques, or therapy, can help support fertility.

- **Can alternative approaches like acupuncture or herbal remedies enhance fertility?**

  While there is limited scientific evidence to support the effectiveness of alternative approaches, some couples have reported positive experiences with practices like acupuncture and certain herbal remedies. It's important to discuss these options with a healthcare professional.

- **How can emotional support be beneficial during the journey of trying to conceive?**

  Struggling with fertility can be emotionally challenging. Joining support groups or seeking counseling and therapy can provide a safe space to share experiences, gain support, and learn coping strategies to navigate the emotional ups and downs.

Have Questions / Comments?

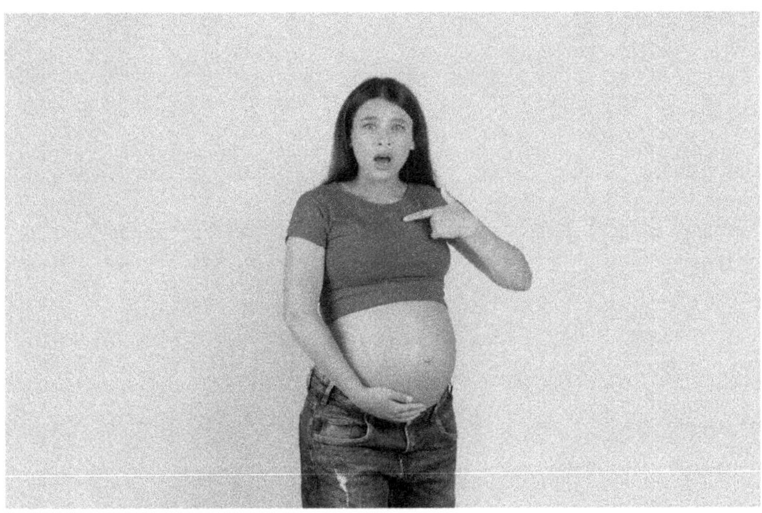

This book was designed to cover as much info as possible but I know I have probably missed something, or some new amazing discovery that has just come out.

If you notice something missing or have a question that I failed to answer, please get in touch and let me know. If I can, I will email you an answer and also update the book so others can also benefit from it.

Thanks For Being Awesome :)

Submit Your Questions / Comments At:

Get How To Be A Super Mom - 100% FREE

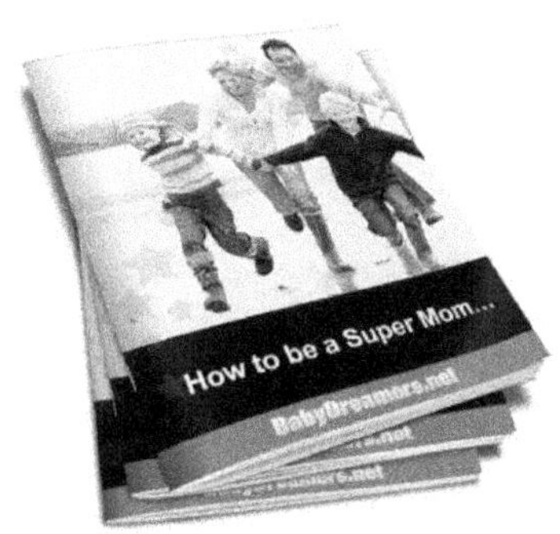

For being one of our amazing readers, we would love to offer you another book we have created, 100% free.

Being a mom is probably the most important job in the world – we've all heard that, and it's true. You're bringing up the next generation of wonderful, intelligent, loving, creative, responsible people.

We all want to be Super Mom and to be everything and do everything, but it this possible?

Being a Super Mom is possible, but you have to learn how to empower yourself to be the kind of Super Mom that you feel you need to be, keeping in mind that the title Super Mom doesn't mean the same thing to everyone.

Get How to be a Super Mom For Free at

BabyDreamers.net